DIETS TO HELP HAY FEVER AND SINUSITIS

25p
net

By the same author

NATUROPATHIC FIRST AID

DIETS TO HELP ASTHMA & BRONCHITIS

DIETS TO HELP

HAY FEVER AND SINUSITIS

by

R. NEWMAN TURNER, N.D., D.O., M.B.N.O.A.

THORSONS PUBLISHERS LIMITED
37/38 Margaret Street, London, W.1.

First published February 1970
Second Impression October 1971

ISBN 0 7225 0158 7

*Made and Printed in Great Britain by
Weatherby Woolnough Ltd., Wellingborough
Northants, England*

CONTENTS

INTRODUCTION

Hay fever and sinusitis are such common complaints nowadays that many people accept them as part of their existence. Together with headaches, constipation and a few other ailments they are regarded as something the sufferer has got to 'learn to live with'. Like a rainy or foggy day, they have to be tolerated and most people believe very little can be done about them. If the symptoms become more than just a nuisance and medical advice is sought there is still no satisfaction, for there is no drug or method of treatment in orthodox medicine that can be said to effect a lasting cure for hay fever and sinusitis.

Possibly one of the reasons for this is the almost total lack of reference to the nutritional aspects of conditions such as hay fever and sinusitis. But thousands of people have successfully overcome these complaints by the adoption of a sound dietetic regime. For many years naturopaths, osteopaths and medical herbalists have helped many sufferers from hay fever and sinus disorders by the use of therapeutic diets in conjunction with physical and biochemical readjustment of body functions.

You might feel that you suffer enough already without inflicting the further discipline of a diet upon yourself. But if you hope to cure your complaint, a degree of dietary control is bound to be necessary at some stage and the sooner you start to use a constructive approach the sooner will you begin to feel better. Dietary therapy need not be unpleasant—it is simply a matter of observing certain basic rules and making an interesting menu within the framework of a sound wholefood regime.

This book in the series is designed to show you the principal dietetic rules for the successful management of hay fever and sinusitis. The main types of food to be avoided, as well as those of which you may need more, are discussed. A maintenance diet, based on the nutritional principles outlined, is given and there are stricter diets for the more intensive treatment of the complaint and management of the acute attacks. The final chapter will give a selection of recipes which contain only those ingredients that would be suitable for your illness.

Our knowledge of dietetics is still very much in its infancy and what information we have is based on clinical experience and a limited amount of research. Our knowledge may, in fact, never be complete, for nutritional requirements vary with every individual, but we know enough to be able to offer hope to the sufferer from acute and chronic hay fever or sinusitis. It is the hope of the author that this series will provide the information which will enable you to adopt a more constructive attitude to your health and to enjoy life more fully.

CHAPTER 1

WHAT HAPPENS IN HAY FEVER AND SINUSITIS?

The answer to that question is all too familiar to the sufferer from either of these complaints. The symptoms affect the face and head, and like most ailments of that part of the body, they dominate the life of the sufferer because they are 'so close to you'. Unlike a pain in the leg, or abdomen, you cannot forget about it for a time.

Hay fever is said to affect only predisposed persons, that is people with an inherited tendency to the complaint. In other words, if your parents or grandparents, or other members of your family, suffer from hay fever or asthma, you may have an inherent susceptibility to the condition. This does not mean that you will inevitably suffer, for the inherited weakness can be overcome.

The symptoms of hay fever are characteristic and sometimes severe. Initially there may be itching of the nose, mouth, pharynx and eyes. Very soon there is a profuse nasal discharge and watering of the eyes. The irritation may cause sneezing. The nasal membranes swell up and, as mucus production becomes greater, there may be nasal congestion which will also affect the sinuses as the illness progresses.

In more sensitive individuals there may even be swelling of the eyes and face and some people will suffer from asthma simultaneously. The latter may already have been asthma sufferers in childhood and as the causes of this are basically similar to those of hay fever it is not surprising that the condition is aggravated when there is a disorder of another part of the respiratory system.

Perhaps it is some consolation for hay fever sufferers that their attacks tend to occur only during the spring and summer. At such times pollens, dust, and fungal spores are more abundant and these are allergens—substances which precipitate attacks in sensitive individuals. Some people, however, may suffer from symptoms similar to hay fever throughout the year and these may often be associated with attacks of sinusitis.

The sufferer from chronic sinusitis is even less fortunate, as his symptoms not only persist throughout the year but may be aggravated both by allergens in the summer months, if he is susceptible to them, and by cold, wet weather in the winter. The pattern of nasal discharge, pain and tenderness over the forehead and cheek bones may occur frequently and between these attacks there is chronic catarrh, obstructed breathing and, as one might expect, where normal air intake is impeded, general debility. In the chronic case the pressure of accumulated catarrh in sinuses already congested by swollen mucous membranes may lead to severe headaches. Catarrh from the nasal passages can also pass down the windpipe and affect the lungs.

Why the symptoms occur

What happens is painfully obvious to the sufferer from either hay fever or sinusitis. Perhaps more important is why it happens and what can be done about it.

To appreciate the mechanisms involved in attacks of hay fever and sinusitis we must know something of the anatomy and normal functions of the affected area, the nasal passages and sinuses. As you inspire air normally it does not go directly from nasal passage to lungs but circulates through the cavities in the facial bones known as the nasal sinuses. There are five pairs of sinus cavities, all connected with the nasal cavity. The largest of these, the frontal sinuses, lie above the bridge of the nose and over the eye sockets on either side. The maxillary sinuses are in the cheek bones. Other sinuses are present in the ethmoid and sphenoid bones of the skull, which are situated behind the other facial bones. Their cavities connect with the nasal cavity and frontal sinuses by small bony apertures.

The sinus cavities help to make the skull lighter and also aid in vocal resonance. They are also believed to perform the same function as the nasal cavity, that of warming and moistening the air we breathe in. The sinuses are lined with mucous membrane similar to that in the nose, and in normal health the secretion by this membrane should be just sufficient to moisten the air and to trap dust particles and other foreign bodies before it passes down to the lungs. It is the integrity of this mucous membrane that is of critical importance in conditions such as hay fever and sinusitis.

When the lining of the sinus cavities becomes irritated it secretes more mucus than normal and may also become inflamed. The narrow apertures through which the mucus normally drains become obstructed and catarrhal congestion ensues, with the possible development of pus. Hard blowing of the nose in an attempt to eliminate the cararrh may aggravate the condition by creating a back pressure leading to further congestion.

In the hay fever sufferer the mucous membrane is more sensitive than in the normal individual and certain external irritants such as pollens or house dust precipitate an attack. These irritants are called allergens.

Allergens

The susceptibility of hay fever sufferers varies. The majority of people have their attacks in spring and summer, when grass pollens are abundant. In certain areas the condition may continue through the autumn, when plants such as ragweed are in flower. But the condition is not, strictly speaking, just 'hay fever' because other allergens, such as tree pollens, house dust, fungus spores, or animal hair, can precipitate an attack.

The reason that these allergens cause such severe irritation and subsequent symptoms is believed to be because they are composed of protein molecules which are larger than those of normal proteins which we absorb from our food. Healthy blood vessels and mucous membranes have a fine closely-knit structure which only allows smaller molecules to penetrate. In individuals showing an allergic reaction, however, the poorer quality of the blood vessel walls and membranes permits the entry of the larger protein molecules which act as irritants. The irritant action of these allergens causes the release from the tissues of a substance called histamine which brings about swelling of mucous membranes. Sometimes the swelling is more widespread once the allergen has entered the blood stream and the eyes and face become puffy. In severe attacks even the extremities may be affected.

Internal irritants, in the form of toxic metabolites, or waste products, can be a causative factor in hay fever and sinusitis. These will bring about a lowered state of resistance of the mucous membranes and give rise to a catarrhal condition which is the forerunner of sinusitis.

Allergens may not be the only cause of swelling of the mucous membranes. There may be structural faults which cause poor drainage and congestion, nasal polyps (small growths which occur in unhealthy tissue), or fibrosis of the apertures resulting from old inflammatory conditions. If there is to be adequate drainage of the sinuses it can be seen how important the growth and development of these structures is in children. They should be taught correct breathing and have adequate chewing of fresh raw food during the developmental years to exercise the jaw muscles and to stimulate the normal growth of the facial bones.

Conventional treatments for hay fever and sinusitis have proved consistently to be ineffective in the long term. Tests to discover specific allergens, and then giving a course of injections to desensitize the individual, seldom have any lasting benefit. Anti-histamines are widely used, but they do no more than alleviate the symptoms of congestion in hay fever. They merely antagonize what is a normal defensive reaction by the body and do nothing to correct the underlying imbalance which has resulted in the release of the histamine in the tissues. Nasal sprays and inhalants are not, of course, considered a cure, but their repeated use can also have a permanently damaging effect on the nasal mucous membranes.

Chronic congestive sinusitis may become so severe that surgical drainage is advocated. This is an unpleasant procedure and, although it may be necessary in severe cases, it is again of no lasting benefit since the condition will return if the fundamental cause is not removed.

It should be obvious from the foregoing description of the mechanism of hay fever and sinus disorders, that constructive therapy is required to increase the resistance of the affected areas and reduce their sensitivity, as well as measures to improve the general health of the sufferer. By tackling the overall condition of the patient and not just treating his local symptoms, a great deal of progress can be achieved, progress of a lasting nature.

One of the most important aspects of these conditions is the nutritional one.

CHAPTER 2

HOW AND WHY DIET CAN HELP

Hay fever and sinusitis sufferers are so often told that their diet will make no difference to their condition. Apart from some work on food allergens, very little attention has been paid to the nutritional aspects of these conditions by orthodox physicians, yet diet is one of the important factors influencing the general health of the sufferer and his susceptibility to develop specific conditions such as those we are considering.

By attention to certain details of the diet it is possible to alleviate a great deal of the distress caused by hay fever and sinusitis. Corrective nutrition is one of the ways of treating the cause of these complaints and by following a balanced dietary programme you will be achieving far more than by the continual use of preparations which give only temporary relief of the symptoms. Symptomatic relief is, of course, often necessary, but it is both useless and harmful if it is relied upon to the exclusion of constructive measures to correct the disordered metabolism which has given rise to the condition. It is far better, in any case, to use a natural herbal or homœopathic substance to alleviate the symptoms, and very often this may prove more effective than the most powerful chemically prepared drugs.

There are three ways in which one's diet can affect hay fever and sinusitis:

(a) By *excess* of foods which can act as irritants, or have a toxic effect resulting in production of more catarrh. Such food items as milk and starches fall in this category. Their harmful effect may be very small but the cumulative action, when taken regularly over a long period, may contribute to the development of the symptoms.

(b) By *deficiency* of various vitamins, minerals and trace elements. This may come about by eating refined foods such as white flour, white sugar and canned or frozen foods, from which much of the nutritional quality has been removed or lost. The regular intake of such foods will result in a deterioration in the tone of the mucous membrane and a general lack of resistance.

(c) By an *allergic reaction.* Apart from the pollens, which have already been discussed, certain foods may cause an allergic reaction part of which may be the symptoms of hay fever. Included in this category are strawberries and shell fish. These foods can only cause an allergic reaction in the individual who is particularly sensitive to them. Not everybody is allergic to these types of foods. Many people, however, may be allergic to a wide variety of other foods without realizing it. The offending food does not have the dramatic and immediate effect on the health that strawberries or shell fish do in susceptible individuals, but if included in the diet over a period of time it may disturb normal health sufficiently to give rise to chronic symptoms for which no other cause can be found. The most satisfactory method of determining which foods are likely to be unsuitable for you is the pulse test.[1]

If you want to overcome your hay fever or sinusitis it can be done with a determined effort to correct dietary errors and by adopting a nutritional regime which will maintain a high level of health.

It is advisable to start by cutting out or reducing all

[1] *The Pulse Test* by Arthur F. Coca, M.D. (Arc Books, New York).

those foods which have a harmful effect in one way or another. Then you should ensure that the diet is well balanced, with adequate proportions of the foods which are particularly necessary to increase resistance and general health against hay fever and sinus disorders.

At some stage, depending on the severity and on how long you have suffered from the complaint, it may be wise to follow a stricter diet, or even carry out short fasts, in order to bring about a better elimination of catarrh and to speed up recovery. This may be necessary in any case when there is an acute attack, for the system is better able to overcome the symptoms when less energy is being used for digestion and it can be made available for the eliminative effort. Instructions on the various stages of dietary treatment are given in the chapters which follow.

Whilst an improvement may be noticeable even a few weeks after starting the new dietary regime, it may take very much longer to overcome a condition such as sinusitis, particularly where you have suffered for many years. Functional and organic changes take place which can only gradually be reversed, and it may take several years of perseverance, during which you may suffer apparent setbacks and aggravations of your symptoms, before the complaint eventually disappears.

The adoption of a dietary plan is a basic essential in the treatment of both hay fever and sinusitis and without doing this there is little hope of permanent recovery. However, diet alone will not be sufficient in the majority of cases. Mechanical factors, affecting the blood supply and nerve supply to nasal passages and sinuses, as well as other important organs such as the liver, may require osteopathic treatment. The balancing of organ function and vitality by acupuncture will certainly be of benefit, or you may require a herbal or homœopathic prescription, to correct body chemistry and improve the tone of the tissues. Even psychological factors should be considered, as both hay fever and sinusitis can frequently be the physical expression of some emotional stress or anxiety.

After introducing your dietary changes, therefore, visit a naturopath, who will be able to advise you on these aspects of your treatment, as well as assessing your more specific nutritional requirements.

CHAPTER 3

SOME FOODS YOU SHOULD AVOID

As mentioned earlier some foods can have an adverse effect upon health by their cumulative action, creating imbalance and deficiency. A direct relationship between the intake of these foods and the onset of hay fever or sinusitis has not yet been proved, but their effect in lowering general health and resistance is quite definite. Some food items may be taken for many years without apparent adverse effects but it is the gradual build-up in the system of certain of their constituents to a level at which they disturb the normal functions of certain organs that is important. The body attempts to neutralize and eliminate any harmful substances that are ingested with our food and symptoms may not become apparent until the burden becomes too great, or there is some disturbance of eliminative functions. These dietary factors, superimposed on constitutional or structural weaknesses, can precipitate your illness.

We will discuss in this chapter some of the more obvious trouble-makers in the average diet which should be avoided altogether, and some of which you should considerably reduce your intake. This does not mean that there will be little left in the diet worth enjoying, for in succeeding chapters we shall consider foods which may be taken and indeed some which are essential to maintain health.

Milk and certain Milk Products

When the cells of the membranes lining the nasal cavities and sinuses are irritated by foreign bodies they secrete mucus as a protective mechanism. Similarly, when an allergen causes the release of histamine in the tissues, and the consequent swelling, mucus is again produced. When mucus production becomes excessive, catarrh is formed. Catarrh consists of protein and carbohydrate and the more foods of that nature taken in the diet, the greater will be the tendency to catarrhal secretions.

Milk consists of protein, fat, and carbohydrate, in almost equal proportions, and whilst it is frequently regarded as a a complete food, it does not seem to be very well assimilated by many people after infancy. This is chiefly because of the structure of the proteins in cows' milk, which are of the type that is tougher and more difficult to digest. The result of a high intake of milk and milk products, such as cheese, is more catarrhal secretion.

Milk, and the harder varieties of cheese, should, therefore, be eliminated from your diet if you are a hay fever or sinusitis sufferer. In hay fever this may not remove the cause, but it goes some way towards alleviating the symptoms by reducing the catarrhal secretion.

Yogurt should also be avoided in the early stages of your treatment and during any acute attacks, although this may be included in a balanced diet at a later stage.

Foods made with milk, such as milk puddings, custards, and blancmanges, and drinks such as cocoa or coffee with milk, should be avoided. A small amount of milk may be taken in tea, provided you do not drink large quantities of tea. In drinks such as tea, or other beverages, it is preferable to use a low fat milk such as soya-milk or a plant milk, both of which are obtainable from health food stores.

Low-fat cream cheeses are permitted and a good quality cottage cheese, or lactic cheese, are better than the harder varieties, and are easier to digest.

One further argument against milk as a food is that

some individuals have been found to be allergic to it. This is not a common allergy but it may exist in a mild form without being very obvious to the sufferer. Sometimes the antibiotics administered to cattle are passed through to the consumer in milk and in many cases this has been thought to be responsible for the development of certain conditions.

Fats and fried foods

Animal fats in the average diet occur chiefly in milk and its derivatives which have already been referred to. They have a high content of saturated fatty-acids and as such they are more difficult to digest than vegetable oils, which are rich in unsaturated fatty-acids, the type which we require to maintain health. The less efficient our fat digestion is, the more likelihood there is of developing gall-bladder disease. The liver and gall-bladder must be functioning at an optimum level if general health and resistance are to be maintained. You should, therefore, reduce the amount of animal fats in your diet and use instead the vegetable oils, such as sunflowerseed oil.

The frying of foods also renders the fats less digestible and this method of cooking is to be avoided in the early stages of your treatment.

Sugar

Sugar, especially refined white sugar, comes high on the list of forbidden foods. While you are treating hay fever and sinusitis you should not take even brown sugar, or sugar substitutes.

Sugar is a toxic irritant which contributes to a wide variety of complaints. It not only acts as an internal irritant to the mucous membranes, but also tends to leach the body's calcium reserves and in this way lowers the general resistance. There is definite evidence to suggest that those who take large amounts of sugar in various forms actually create a chronic state of low blood-sugar level. Low blood-sugar means less vitality and poor resistance to disease.

Foods which contain sugar must also be avoided or reduced in quantity. Cakes, biscuits, proprietary puddings, canned fruit and, of course, sweets and chocolates, all contain added sugar (or artificial sweeteners, which have much the same effect) and these must be eliminated from the diet.

Natural sugar, which is better assimilated, and provides all the body's energy requirements, may be taken in the form of honey, dried fruits, and grapes. These contain minerals and trace elements which are required in our diet whereas refined sugar does not. A good quality honey should always be used when a sweetener is required. Some authorities suggest that honey is of specific benefit in cases of hay fever and sinusitis.

Starches

The same restriction applies to the starchy foods as to sugar. All starches are reduced to sugar during digestion and, if the intake is excessive, their ultimate effect is similar.

Bread, especially that made with white flour, pastry, cakes, biscuits and bananas should be reduced or even avoided altogether. Moderate amounts of wholemeal bread, or brown rye biscuits, or pumpernickel, are permitted, except when on a strict eliminative diet. As a general rule any starchy food in the diet should be in the minor proportion.

Stimulants

Under this heading come such items as coffee, strong tea, alcohol, tobacco and spices. Whilst no direct cause or relationship has been established between, say, coffee drinking and hay fever or sinusitis, the caffeine present in the beverage does have an adverse effect on general health, disturbing, in particular, the functions of the liver and gall-bladder. The liver is responsible for the break-down of all impurities in our food to a form which can be eliminated. When there is disturbance of liver function the level of toxic substances in the blood rises and there is, consequently, a great burden upon the mucous linings of the sinus and nasal cavities.

You would, therefore, be wise to avoid drinking coffee regularly. Use instead a decaffeinated coffee, or better still a coffee substitute or other beverage, which can be obtained from a health food store.

The same restriction applies to tea, to a lesser degree, and to alcohol which also has a high sugar content. China tea is better in general than the Indian variety.

Table salt should not be used, either as a condiment or in cooking. Salt tends to cause fluid retention in the tissues. Prolonged cooking of vegetables in salt also causes a loss of many of the vitamins and minerals naturally present. The only type of salt permitted, for cooking if necessary or at the table, is sea salt, obtainable from a health food store.

Meat and fish

It is not the purpose of this booklet to advocate vegetarianism, although this is undoubtedly a healthier type of diet for the majority of people. Meat is not well digested and causes a high level of impurities in the system, and if you are not already a vegetarian it is certainly advisable to reduce the amount of meat that is eaten. For many people, however, it would be unwise to make a sudden change to a vegetarian diet as this may create problems of readjustment. As the hay fever and sinusitis sufferer should reduce the intake of the dairy proteins, some meat and fish may be desirable as an alternative to these.

Whatever meat is eaten should be of the lean varieties. Fish is preferable as this provides a higher content of vitamins A and D, and is generally more readily digested.

CHAPTER 4

SOME FOODS YOU REQUIRE

Most of the foods referred to in the previous chapter can be avoided altogether, or reduced considerably, and the stricter one is about this the greater will be the improvement in health. There are, however, many foods which you must include in a balanced diet to maintain a high level of health and resistance to disease.

Such foods should be rich in their content of vitamins, minerals and trace elements, and one way of ensuring this is to eat foods as near their natural state as possible. Always try to select foods which have been grown naturally, without the use of artificial fertilizers and chemical pesticides. The best way of ensuring that your food has been naturally grown and prepared with the minimum loss of nutritional value is to shop at a health food store. The produce available there is selected because it has not undergone the considerable refinement, and removal of nutrients found in the natural state, that is the case with many mass-produced foodstuffs nowadays.

The two most important vitamins required by sufferers from hay fever and sinusitis are vitamins A and C.

Vitamin A is found chiefly in the form of carotene, a precursor of the vitamin, present in vegetables and some dairy foods, such as eggs. Carotene is fat-soluble, which means that a sufficiency of unsaturated fatty-acids must be available for it to be converted into vitamin A in our bodies. It is, therefore, necessary to use vegetable oils, such as corn oil, or sunflower-seed oil. Adequate supplies of vitamin A are essential to the health of skin, hair and mucous membranes, and to increase resistance to infection. The principal vegetable sources of carotene are shown in Table 1.

TABLE 1

CAROTENE CONTENT OF VEGETABLES AND FRUITS

FOOD	CAROTENE I.U./100g.
Carrots, mature	20,000
Spinach	13,000
Carrots, young	10,000
Cress	8,000
Watercress	5,000
Apricot	2,000
Lettuce	2,000
Tomato	1,200
Brussels sprouts	700
Cabbage	500

The adequate utilization of *vitamin C* also depends on the presence of vitamin A. Vitamin C is important to increase resistance to infection, and it also has an anti-allergic reaction. It is, therefore, necessary in abundance in the diet of hay fever sufferers. Table 2 shows the principal vitamin C-rich foods. It will be noted that vegetables are, in many cases, richer sources than some fruits.

Fruit and Vegetables

From the above it will be seen that these should form the greater proportion of the diet, and preferably they

TABLE 2

FOOD SOURCES OF VITAMIN C

FOOD	VITAMIN C Mg./100g. approx.
Fruits	
Apples	4.60
Blackberries, raw	21.00
Grapefruit	40.00
Guava	300.00
Melon	32.00
Orange	49.30
Strawberries	60.00
Raspberries	24.00
Blackcurrants	57.00
Vegetables	
Cabbage, raw	78.00
French beans	14.00
Tomato, raw	23.00
Watercress, raw	80.00

should be taken in the raw state. Almost any type of fruit or vegetable may be eaten, except some soft fruits to which you may be allergic. Bananas should be avoided, however, because of their high starch content.

Vegetables and fruit provide nourishment and energy with little or no toxic effect upon the system. They are rich in many of the vitamins and minerals we require, particularly vitamins A and C, which are essential for the normal functions of the mucous membranes.

Fruits also provide natural sugar for energy. Dried

fruits are particularly valuable in this respect and should be included in the diet in place of sugar and other sweeteners.

It is important to ensure that your daily menu contains a generous proportion of some of those fruits or vegetables shown in Tables 1 and 2, which are rich sources of vitamins A and C.

Proteins

Although it is important to avoid the excessive intake of certain types of protein these are, none the less, an important part of the balanced diet. They are essential to provide heat and energy for the body, and the best forms in which to take them are the vegetable proteins, such as the pulses, cereal grains and nuts.

You should, therefore, use such vegetables as beans, peas, lentils and soya products. The cereal grains, such as millet, buckwheat and brown rice may be used as these also have a relatively high protein content.

Nuts are an excellent source of protein, and with few exceptions, nut kernels contain between 12 per cent and 15 per cent. (It is also worth noting that walnuts have a vitamin C content which compares very favourably with other sources, such as orange juice or rose hip syrup.) Nuts should, therefore, be included in the balanced diet and may form the basis of savoury dishes, or be ground and sprinkled over fruit or other desserts.

Carbohydrates

Carbohydrates are also necessary as energy foods. The vegetable carbohydrates should form the greater proportion of the diet. Any cereals in the diet should be of the whole grain type, such as millet, buckwheat, rice and whole wheat.

CHAPTER 5

THE BASIC DIET

If you are not accustomed to what is known as a food reform diet and the nutritional approach to hay fever and sinusitis is new to you, you may find it difficult to make a complete change immediately. The transition from a conventional diet to a healthier, more balanced one is best made gradually.

The adjustment by the body to a rapid change in eating habits may often precipitate some unpleasant minor symptoms, which are relatively harmless in themselves and may, indeed, be an indication that the body is responding by the elimination of toxic encumbrances. Such episodes are familiar to natural therapy practitioners, being termed 'healing crises' or 'aggravations'. Normally they should be allowed to take their course, but if in doubt you should obtain the professional advice of a naturopath or medical herbalist. However, severe aggravations can generally be avoided by making a gradual transition to a balanced, health-gaining diet.

The basic diet is one which contains all the food constituents that are necessary to maintain good health and to bring about an improvement in the sufferer from specific disorders, such as hay fever and sinusitis. It will also serve as a transition towards the stricter diets that may be necessary for the treatment of these conditions, details of which are given in the chapter which follows.

If you only suffer mildly from either hay fever or sinusitis, a change to the basic diet may be all that is required to achieve a considerable improvement. If the conditions are more severe then it may be essential to undergo the stricter diets. It will certainly be necessary to follow the basic diet for some weeks, even if there is a rapid improvement in your condition, as to abandon it too soon would almost inevitably invite a recurrence of the complaint. This type of diet can, in fact, be followed indefinitely and if you suffer from chronic sinusitis or have suffered from hay fever for many years, it may well take several years of dietary and other measures to eradicate these complaints completely. However, the improvement in general health and well being after following a diet such as that which is given makes the more specific problems which arise much easier to tackle, and other forms of treatment are more effective when the basic obstructions have been removed and a better resistance developed by sound nutrition.

The basic diet outlined here gives a number of alternatives for each meal, all of which take into consideration the requirements referred to in the foregoing chapters. The emphasis of any diet for catarrhal conditions, such as sinusitis, must be upon fresh fruit and vegetables. The better the quality of these the more valuable they will be nutritionally, and for this reason you should always try to obtain organically grown produce.

To ensure that your foods are naturally grown and prepared it is better to shop at a health food store, although even there you should read the labels carefully before buying, as some products contain substances which might not be suitable for your complaint.

Try to eat as much food as possible in the raw state, and you should always endeavour to start a meal with some raw fruit or salad. When cooking vegetables or fruit, do it only long enough to make the food tender. They should be cooked in only a small quantity of water, without salt being added, for a short time. In this way the vitamin losses are minimal.

Further details as to preparation of foods and recipes will be found in Chapter 7.

Menu

On rising

Drink of freshly extracted orange, pineapple or apple juice, or warm water with lemon juice and honey. If fresh extraction of juices is not possible use bottled or canned, pure unsweetened juices obtainable from a health food store or high-class grocer.

Breakfast

For those who take very little breakfast, or none at all, but like to have something to drink, the following are recommended:

Pure fruit juices or vegetable juices as above, or a special drink (see page 47), weak China tea with lemon or a little milk (a soya-milk substitute, or Plamil, are recommended, but a small amount of cow's milk in tea is permitted at this stage), a cereal beverage or coffee substitute.

To eat, choose from the following, according to appetite:

Whole nuts with raisins.

Soaked, dried apricots or prunes, or other dried fruits as available.

Fresh fruit, or fruit salad made from apples, pears, grapes, oranges, peaches, plums, melon, etc., as available.

Puréed or grated apple, with wheatgerm and raisins.

Stewed or baked apple with wheatgerm or raisins.

Muesli (see page 47).

A small portion of pure goat's milk yogurt may be taken with the fruit dishes at breakfast.

Two or 3 slices brown rye biscuit, Vita Wheat, pumpernickel, or wholemeal toast, with a little butter or sunflower oil margarine, and savoury spread or honey.

Mid-morning

Warm drinks: coffee substitute, weak tea, or savoury drink, e.g. Barmene, Vecon or Marmite—one teaspoonful in a cup of hot water.

Cold drinks: pure fruit or vegetable juice.

Do not eat.

Mid-day meal

Small glass of freshly extracted vegetable juice as an apéritif, or a serving of single or mixed vegetable soup.

Large or small combination salad, according to appetite. A portion of cheese or milled nuts or dried fruit may be taken with the salad, or you may have a serving of a savoury, such as a millet or nut dish, or a potato baked in its jacket with a little vegetable oil. One or two slices of pumpernickel, or rye bread, or wholemeal bread may be taken, with a little butter or sunflower oil margarine and a savoury spread, if desired, with the salad.

Dessert: fresh or dried fruit, using only honey or maple syrup for sweetening, if required. Fruit jelly. Gelozone or carrageen mould. Egg custard. Muesli.

Milled nuts or wheatgerm may be added to a fruit or vegetable salad.

Afternoon

Drinks as for mid-morning. It is preferable not to eat, but if you are accustomed to having something, one or two wholemeal biscuits or some fresh fruit may be taken.

Evening Meal

Fruit or vegetable juice apéritif, or vegetable soup (if not already taken at lunchtime).

Savoury dish with one or two conservatively cooked vegetables. Mixed vegetable stew. Combination salad as at mid-day meal.

Dessert: Fresh or dried fruit or fruit jelly as at mid-day meal.

On Retiring

Drink of fruit or vegetable juice, or warm drink of cereal beverage made with water and a little milk substitute, or other drink as desired.

Do not eat.

Note: The mid-day and evening meals may be transposed if desired, or you may have a combination salad at both meals instead of a warm dish. It is preferable to have one salad meal per day. If it is difficult to have this type of menu for your mid-day meal while you are at work, you should either take fresh fruit, or sandwiches made with wholemeal bread or biscuits, or have the cooked meal at mid-day and the salad meal in the evening.

CHAPTER 6

STRICT DIETS FOR HAY FEVER AND SINUSITIS

When you have followed the balanced diet for some weeks, you may feel able to undertake a short, stricter diet to increase elimination.

Strict dietary measures are certainly necessary if you suffer from any aggravation of the symptoms, which may occur after you have been on the balanced diet for some time. This aggravation can be regarded as an encouraging sign—an indication that a greater eliminative effort is being made by the body. Chronic sinusitis sufferers accumulate a great deal of mucus and purulent catarrh which obstructs the respiratory passages. Once this starts to come away, perhaps in the form of a heavy cold, it is necessary to eat only very lightly, to enable the catarrh to be eliminated without further mucus production.

If you have hay fever you may, of course, suffer aggravations due to a raised pollen count, or exposure to some other allergen. This type of attack requires herbal or homœopathic medication, but it will be of assistance to keep to a low carbohydrate, low protein diet to minimize mucus secretion.

People in whom the conditions of hay fever or sinusitis have been long-standing, or are particularly severe, may find it necessary to repeat the strict diet a number of times. If there is not a definite improvement when this is done, however, do not lose hope, for chronic conditions require 'chronic treatment' and it may well take several years of perseverance during which time your complaint will become gradually less severe and troublesome.

There are two types of strict diet for hay fever or sinusitis, the short-term cleansing diet, and the longer strict diet. The short cleansing diet is suitable for hay fever sufferers, and can be repeated at intervals of three to four weeks, or as required. This diet will also be of benefit to those sufferers from sinusitis who are unable to undertake the longer strict diet because of restrictions imposed by work or time. Long-standing sinusitis will, however, require strict dietary treatment at some stage if it is to be satisfactorily cured. The longer strict diet has a greater eliminative stimulus to the body, but it is not wise to undertake it without the advice and guidance of a naturopathic practitioner unless you are accustomed to food reform diets of this type.

MODIFIED CLEANSING DIET

First two days

Fresh fruit only. Any kind of fruit except bananas, rhubarb, plums, gooseberries. The fruit may be eaten raw or cut up into a fruit salad. If fruit salad is made use only a little honey for sweetening, otherwise omit the fruit if it cannot be eaten without further sweetening.

Drinks during these two days may consist of fresh pure (or bottled, unsweetened) fruit or vegetable juices, although it is unlikely that much will be required to drink as adequate liquid occurs naturally in the fruit.

Third and fourth days

On rising: Drink of lemon juice with warm water and honey.

Breakfast: Fresh fruit as before, or baked or puréed apples, with raisins.

Between meals: Fruit juice or savoury drink, e.g.,

Marmite, Barmene, or Vecon—one teaspoonful in a cup of hot water.

Lunch: Raw combination salad with dried fruit and dressing if desired. No savoury or biscuits are to be taken with the salad at this stage.

Fresh fruit for dessert.

Evening meal: Raw salad again as for lunch.

Fresh or soaked dried fruit for dessert.

On retiring: Fruit juice, or savoury drink.

Fifth to Seventh days

On rising: Lemon or apple cider vinegar drink (see recipes).

Breakfast: Fresh fruit, or soaked dried prunes or apricots, or baked or stewed or puréed apples. Raisins or wheatgerm may be added to the fruit if desired.

Lunch: Raw combination salad. A portion of milled nuts may now be added, or some wheatgerm may be sprinkled on the salad. Small portion of lactic or cottage cheese may be taken.

Fresh or dried fruit for dessert.

Evening meal: Raw salad as before, or mixed vegetable broth, or two or three conservatively cooked vegetables, served with a light egg dish, or a little steamed fish, or a vegetable casserole (see recipes).

On retiring: Fruit juice or savoury drink as before.

Note: The mid-day and evening meals may be transposed if desired. If you are away from home during the day and find it difficult to obtain a meal as described, then you should take fresh fruit, with some nuts and raisins.

This diet may be extended for a further week by continuing to follow the directions for the fifth to seventh days, or you may return to the balanced diet given in the previous chapter.

STRICT CLEANSING DIET

Important note: Unless you have been accustomed to a food reform diet, containing a high proportion of fruit and vegetables, for some time, you should not attempt to follow this diet without obtaining professional advice from a naturopath. Whilst it will be of great benefit to the majority of sufferers from hay fever and sinusitis, some people may not be constitutionally suited to such a diet, and even those who are may experience aggravations, or 'healing crises'. These are often a good sign but you should be guided through them by a practitioner who understands the various stages of recovery. You should also endeavour to rest as much as possible during the first week or two of the diet.

First week

Days 1 *and* 2: Fast, taking only pure water or fruit or vegetable juices. One tumblerful of juice may be taken four to five times daily according to thirst. Any kind of fresh fruit juice may be used, such as apple, orange, grape, or vegetable juice, such as carrot, celery, or beetroot. The juices should, if possible, be freshly extracted. The vegetable juices can be mixed or combinations may be taken—carrot and apple juice are a good combination for sinusitis sufferers.

If fresh juices are unobtainable the bottled or canned fruit or vegetable juices may be used, but these should be pure and free of any sweeteners or other additives. Never use 'soft drinks' or squashes, such as the popular brands which have 'added glucose'.

If you prefer a hot drink one of the brands of pure, concentrated apple juices may be taken with warm water, or a savoury drink may be made using Marmite, Barmene or Vecon (one teaspoonful in a cup of hot water).

Days 3 *to* 5: Fresh fruit only. Any kind of fruit except

rhubarb or bananas, and certain soft fruits (e.g. plums, gooseberries). Take as much of the fruit as appetite demands, at mealtimes. If preferred fruit can be cut up or grated to make a fruit salad, with a little honey for sweetening if necessary.

For those who, for various reasons, find raw fruit unpalatable or indigestible, it may be puréed or stewed and eaten thus with the addition of some raisins and a little honey for sweetening.

If drinks are required between meals you may take fruit juices or savoury drinks as before, or weak China tea with lemon or a dash of plant- or soya-milk.

Days 6 *and* 7*:* Breakfast: Fresh fruit juice, or lemon and honey drink. Fresh or dried fruit.

Between meals: One small glassful freshly extracted carrot juice, or mixed fruit or vegetable drink, or warm drink (e.g. weak tea, cereal coffee, etc.).

Lunch: Raw combination salad (see recipes), with dressing, or, clear vegetable broth.

Fresh fruit as dessert.

Evening meal: As for lunch.

Second week: Breakfast: Pure fruit juice drink.

Fresh or dried fruit. If made into a fruit salad a little wheatgerm and honey or maple syrup may be added.

For warm drink, if desired, weak China tea or cereal coffee, or herbal tea may be taken (especially peppermint, verbena, or linseed teas).

Between meals: fresh cool fruit or vegetable drink as above, or warm drink as above.

Mid-day meal: Raw salad as above, but you may now add dried fruit and milled nuts and a little cottage or lactic cheese, or mixed vegetable soup or broth.

Fresh or dried fruit as dessert.

Evening meal: Raw salad as above, or vegetable soup, or two to three conservatively cooked vegetables in casserole, with a savoury sauce (see recipes) on top.

Fresh fruit or natural fruit jelly or Gelozone or carrageen mould.

Third week: Breakfast: As second week. You may now have a small portion of goat's milk yogurt with the fruit.

Mid-day meal: As second week, but you may now take a slice of wholemeal bread, or one or two slices rye biscuit or pumpernickel with the salad or soup. Apply butter or sunflower oil margarine thinly.

Evening meal: Salad again if desired.

Or savoury protein dish with conservatively cooked vegetables.

Fourth week:

Continuation of fruit and wheatgerm breakfast is desirable. You may now have one or two slices of rye biscuit or wholemeal bread or pumpernickel with sunflower oil margarine or a little butter. Honey should be used rather than other preserves, or you may have a savoury spread.

Of the remaining meals, one should consist entirely of raw salad and fruit, and the other of conservatively cooked vegetables with lean meat, fish, egg, or other savoury dishes. For desserts try to keep to fresh or dried fruit or fruit-based dishes, or biscuits and lactic or cream cheese.

After completing the four weeks of the strict diet you should return to the balanced diet. It is essential to continue to avoid acid-forming foods or drinks, especially those foods which you are warned against in chapter 3.

During the time that you are on the diet it is important to ensure regular, easy bowel action, and if necessary this may be done during the fasting stage by means of a small warm water enema. At any other time only a herbal bowel regulator should be used. The type which swells in the bowel stimulating normal muscular action of the colon is most suitable. Carry out the physical measures, such as hydrotherapy and exercises during this time to improve eliminative functions, oxygenation and general health.

CHAPTER 7

RECIPES

The following recipes and instructions for preparation of foods are selected with the specific requirements of the hay fever and sinusitis patient. All the items given may be taken in the balanced diet without fear of taking excessive amounts of foods which are harmful in any way. Certain items may, however, have to be avoided when on the stricter diets and these will be indicated in the specific diet.

A selection of basic recipes in the different categories are given. For further variety the reader is referred to some of the many excellent recipe books of vegetarian and food reform dishes now available. When using other recipes bear in mind the limitations imposed on the intake of certain foods during the early stages of your treatment.

Soups

It is useful to prepare a vegetable stock which can be used when required. Keep the water in which the vegetables have been cooked and use this in soups or savoury dishes. Savoury spreads such as Marmite, Barmene, or Vecon can be used as stock where it is not possible to make some from fresh vegetables. The spread is mixed in hot water in the desired strength.

Mixed vegetable soup

Selection of any vegetables in season such as carrots, celery, cabbage, cauliflower, beetroot, leeks, tomatoes, onions, lentils, beans, peas, spinach, potatoes.

Five tablespoons sunflower-seed oil. Two tablespoons wholemeal or soya flour. Sea salt. Herbs to flavour.

Sauté chopped onions in sunflower-seed oil. Add wholemeal flour (this can be mixed in half portion with soya flour if desired). Dilute with vegetable stock. Add conservatively cooked vegetables and allow to simmer for ten minutes. Add Barmene, Vecon or Marmite, sea salt and herbs to flavour.

Clear vegetable broth

Vegetable stock, sunflower-seed oil—one dessertspoonful. Barmene, Vecon, etc. to flavour, sea salt and parsley, chives or mint. The vegetable stock is heated and poured over the other ingredients. Allow to simmer for five minutes before serving.

Carrot soup

Two large carrots, one onion, one tablespoonful wholemeal flour, two oz. sunflower oil margarine (or vegetable oil), one teaspoon thyme or other herbs to flavour, one and a half pints water, sea salt.

Dice carrots; peel and chop onion; sauté in margarine or oil with herbs for five minutes. Stir in flour and add water. Cook gently for thirty minutes. Season with sea salt, or add Barmene for flavour.

Onion soup

One tablespoon sunflower seed or corn oil, two large onions, five tablespoons wholemeal flour, four pints of water, sea salt, savoury spreads for flavour, herbs.

Sauté onion in vegetable oil until tender. Add and mix flour. Add vegetable stock and sea salt. Cook thirty to forty-five minutes. Sieve if desired, and serve with the addition of savoury spreads for flavour.

Salads

Combination Salad 1

Half a lettuce, watercress, cress, cucumber, two tomatoes, spring onions, two medium carrots, mint or parsley, milled nuts, St. Ivel lactic cheese.

Break lettuce into bowl. Add watercress, sliced cucumber, tomatoes, and grated carrots. Garnish with mint and parsley and add spring onions. Sprinkle milled nuts over the salad. Serve with lactic cheese and sunflower oil or salad dressing.

Combination salad 2

Half a head of green cabbage, two medium carrots, two onions, lettuce, radishes.

Chop finely the cabbage, radishes, carrots. Serve on bed of lettuce with dressing.

Cabbage salad

Quarter head of red or white cabbage, two onions, two medium carrots, watercress, raisins.

Shred cabbage, watercress and carrots and mix with the raisins. Add sliced onions. Serve with salad dressing.

Winter salad

Half head of cabbage, two to three medium carrots, half raw beetroot, celery, one green pepper, one onion, chicory, nuts, raisins, small portion Cheddar cheese.

Chop or dice the cabbage, celery, pepper, and onion. Grate the carrots and beetroot. Mix all ingredients together in a bowl and add milled nuts and raisins. Break chicory on top and sprinkle dressing over salad before serving.

Apple and vegetable salad

One apple, celery stalks, lettuce leaves or endive, cucumber, nuts.

Chop the celery, endive and cucumber. Mix in bowl rubbed with garlic cloves. Add apple slices and sprinkle with milled nuts. Serve with salad dressing.

Salad Dressings

Lemon and honey dressing

Corn or sunflower seed oil, pure lemon juice or apple cider vinegar, one teaspoonful runny honey, herbs, sea salt.

Mix seventy-five per cent corn or sunflower seed oil with twenty-five per cent lemon juice or cider vinegar, add honey and mix in. Add herbs and sea salt to flavour.

Yogurt dressing

Two to three tablespoonfuls yogurt, lemon juice, onion or garlic, mixed fresh or dried herbs.

Add few drops of lemon juice to the yogurt and chopped onion or garlic and whisk thoroughly together with mixed herbs.

Savoury Dishes

Savoury grains

Whole cereal grains such as millet, buckwheat, rye or brown rice may be used as a savoury dish.

Place the grains in a saucepan and just cover with water. Bring to boil, replace lid and allow to simmer for five to ten minutes, or longer according to the grain. The water should be almost absorbed by the grains. Add grated cheese, chopped onions or mushrooms and flavour with Vecon or Barmene if desired. Serve with salads, or as main dish with two or three conservatively cooked vegetables.

Lentil savoury

Eight oz. lentils, two large onions, three tablespoonfuls sunflower seed oil or corn oil, five to six peeled tomatoes, six oz. grated cheese, one large can soya beans (or fresh soya beans which have been soaked for twenty-four hours in water).

Cook lentils in a little water (just sufficient to cover them) until the water is absorbed. Place in an oven-proof dish. Chop onions and sauté in three tablespoonfuls of vegetable oil. Add soya beans, tomatoes and onions to the lentils. Spread grated cheese over top. Bake in moderate oven for twenty minutes or until cheese is browned.

Stuffed marrow

One medium-sized marrow, two large onions, mushrooms, vegetable oils, one tablespoonful wholemeal flour, quarter pint of water, one egg, four oz. hazel nuts, four oz. bread crumbs, sea salt, sage or mint. Peel and chop the onion. Wash and chop mushrooms and sauté both in vegetable oil. Mix in the other ingredients and cook for two to three minutes. Add sea salt to taste. Cut marrow in half lengthwise and remove skin and seeds. Stuff with the nut mixture, and put halves together again, securing if necessary by wrapping in greaseproof or foil. Place marrow in tin to which a little oil has been added. Cook in moderate oven for forty-five minutes to one hour until marrow is tender. Serve with apple sauce, vegetables or savoury grains.

Mushroom and tomato savoury

Eight oz. breadcrumbs, eight oz. milled nuts. Four

tablespoonfuls vegetable oil, eight oz. mushrooms, eight oz. tomatoes, sea salt, herbs to flavour.

Sauté breadcrumbs and milled nuts in vegetable oil, stirring frequently till crisp. Chop the mushrooms and quarter the tomatoes. Sauté these in vegetable oil for five minutes. Place a little oil in an oven-proof dish and fill with alternate layers of the mushroom mixture and the nut mixture, adding a little sea salt to each layer and herbs if used. Top layer should be nut and breadcrumb mixture. Bake for thirty minutes in a moderate oven. Serve with selection of vegetables.

Baked soya bean savoury

One lb. soya beans, two celery stalks, one tomato, two tablespoonfuls black molasses or runny honey, two quarts water, one onion, one green pepper, garlic or onion to flavour, vegetable oil, pure lemon juice.

If using fresh soya beans, soak overnight in water to which lemon juice has been added, then boil for two hours, or until tender and pour off excess water. Otherwise use canned soya beans from a health food store. Chop celery, onion, pepper and cut up tomato and mix with soya beans. Bake in hot oven for twenty-five minutes. Add a little oil and herbs for flavouring before serving.

Desserts

Fruit compote

Dried apricots, raisins, other fresh fruit in season.

Soak the apricots in half a pint of water overnight with the raisins. Simmer for fifteen minutes. Add fresh fruit suitably chopped or grated. Cook for five minutes and serve with milled nuts or almond cream. Sweeten with runny honey if desired.

Baked apple

Large apple, seedless raisins, two tablespoonfuls milled nuts.

Core the apple. Fill the centre with raisins. Place in a baking dish in a little water. Bake for thirty minutes. Serve with milled nuts sprinkled on top, and runny honey to sweeten if desired.

Stuffed pears

Four pears, almond cream, one tablespoonful each of raisins, sliced pineapple, ground walnuts or almonds.

Halve pears and scoop out cores. Whip almond cream and fold in with raisins, pineapple and milled nuts and place in centre of fruit. Serve with runny honey or maple syrup as desired.

Orange wobbles

One to two cups of pure orange juice, one small teaspoonful agar-agar or portion of pre-prepared carrageen, runny honey.

Whisk agar-agar into about half the orange juice and add the honey. Heat slowly over a gentle heat until the agar-agar is dissolved (do not allow to boil). Add the remaining orange juice and mix. Pour into individual bowls and leave in a cool place to set. Serve with a sprinkling of milled nuts or almond cream.

Apple purée

Two lb. of apples approximately, one cup of apple juice or water, runny honey, lemon peel or cinnamon, milled nuts.

Prepare apples and cut into pieces and cook in apple juice or a little water until tender. Rub through a sieve or prepare in a liquidizer. Mix in honey and lemon peel or cinnamon. Sprinkle with milled nuts and place under grill to brown before serving.

Muesli

Soak organically grown crushed oats in water overnight. Approximately four cupfuls of water to one cupful of crushed oats will be required.

In the morning add one teaspoonful of pure lemon juice and grated apple and any other fresh or dried fruit as desired. The muesli may be served with molasses, fruit juice, wheatgerm, milled nuts or almond cream.

Drinks

Savoury drinks

Savoury drinks may be made from low-sodium Barmene, Marmite, or Vecon. One teaspoonful should be mixed in a cup of hot water.

Cider vinegar and molasses

Mix together one tablespoonful apple cider vinegar and one tablespoonful molasses with warm water.

Lemon and molasses

Mix together one tablespoonful pure lemon juice with one tablespoonful of molasses and hot water.

Lemon and honey

Prepare as above, using runny honey instead of molasses.

Herb teas

These may be obtained in tisanes from a health food store, or the dried herb may be used. If the latter method is used, prepare by pouring boiling water over the herb and allow to steep for five to ten minutes. In the case of linseed tea, one tablespoonful of linseed to one pint of water should be used and this should be boiled for seven to ten minutes and then allowed to steep before straining.

Vegetable juices

These should be freshly extracted in a juicer whenever possible otherwise the pure bottled variety may be used, including the lacto-fermented type. Juices may be taken singly or mixed together. Carrot and apple juice are of particular benefit for hay fever and sinusitis sufferers.